# THE PREGNANT MOM

## DR. WILLIAM RUDOLF

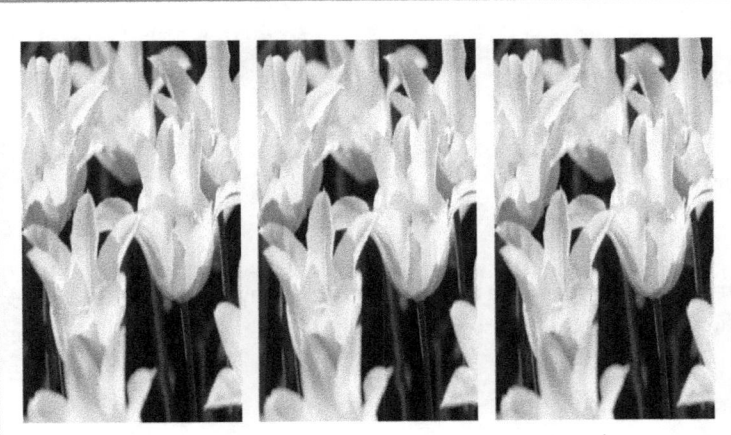

V2C Networks is a company incorporated in the united kingdom having its registered office in London.

Registered company number: 2371917

Published by V2C NETWORKS 2017

ISBN 13:978-1977967565

COPYRIGHT NOTICE

All rights reserved. No part of this publication may be reproduced in any form or by any means (including photocopy or storing it in any medium by electronic means and whether or not transiently or incidentally to some other use of this publication) without the written permission of the copyright owner, except in accordance with the provisions of the copyright, designs and patent act 1988 or under the terms of the licence issued by the copyright licencing agency. Applications for the copyright owner's written permission should be addressed to the publisher via email- bestsellingbooks.com.ng@gmail.com

Typeset by Francis Ortega

Cover design by Tony Ife

Printed by Createspace, an amazon.com company

## DEDICATION

I dedicate this book to the health and life of all babies in this world and to their parents and would-be parents of those still in the belly.

# ACKNOWLEDGMENT

I Want to use this opportunity to thank the owners of www.babycenter.co.uk for their immense contribution and support to this project.

I will also thank Dr. Frigesund for having the time to review this book.

I also want to acknowkedge the contributions of Dr. Williams of the Royal institute of obstetrics and gynaecology in the UK.

I will not forget the contributions of Dr. Isaac Moses for providing some of the pictures used in this project.

I also want to acknowledge the assistance of my secretary, Mrs. Sophia for the numerous times I demanded a good job, thank you.

For every other person that I have failed to mention on this page, please I acknowledge your contributions, thank you very much.

## TABLE OF CONTENTS

1. Mothercare tips during pregnancy
2. Mothercare after childbirth
3. Your body after birth
4. When it is not safe to exercise during pregnancy
5. How to tackle fever safely during pregnancy
6. When you have a still-born
7. Prevention and treatment of diaper rash
8. Developing healthy sleeping habits
9. Great tips on baby feeding
10. How to hold and cradle a baby
11. The best ways to store breast-milk
12. How and when to introduce solid food
13. What to do when your baby chokes
14. If your child begins to vomit
15. How to ease the distress of teething
16. How to handle your baby's hiccups
17. When it is important to see the doctor
18. Dealing with allergies

19  How to bath your baby safely

20  Does your baby have eczema?

21  When your baby cries too much

22  When your baby has cold sores

23  Immunizing your baby

24  Treating insect bites

25  Treatment of skin rashes

26  Bonding with your baby after birth

27  Guides when taking over the counter medicines

28  Other factors to consider during pregnancy

# *INTRODUCTION*

A lot of things come into play when parents make the decision to have a baby . The decisions involves who is going to take care of the child most importantly during the early stages of his development.

You have carried your baby for nine months and has survived the ordeal, so what next?

Eventhough there are many ways to solve this dilemma. Some parents choose use full time child-care while others choose to have one parent stay at home while the other work full time or part time as the case may be.

Whatever your option is, there are basic things you need to learn as a parent in order to give the best care to your child or children during and after delivery.

This book will teach new moms the basics of how to care for your babies eventhough you had no clue about child care and in no time will make you feel like an expert.

This book will teach and inform parents and would-be parents on child care tips during and after pregnancy.

It is very important for parents to have sound knowledge about new born babies and infant care in general.

This book provides all the information all the frequently asked questions on baby eyes, their cries, the mother's breast milk and the importance to the babies and many more information. All the information is broken down in simple language and can be easily understood.

# 1
# MOTHERCARE TIPS DURING PREGNANCY

It is very important that pregnant women adhere too these tips to take care of themselves and the babies they carry. These tips may look so simple but they are very important for they benefit of would-be mothers.

These tips include but not limited to the following;

- In the early stages of pregnancy, you may start feeling weak and tired because your mind is over-working. You might also experience that you are visiting the restroom more frequently. The best thing to do at this stage is to rest during the day whenever you can. Rest is very important at this stage.
- Drink plenty of water and fluids to avoid being dizzy.
- At this stage, it is common to go off or get irritated by certain smells and food. So this are normal, try to avoid such foods and smells which may

- make you want to throw-up.
- You might also be experiencing stomach cramps which may be easily seen as periods.
- You can also be moody most times. So look for events that would engage you and make you happy.
- Certain foods will not be good for a developing baby like alcohol, caffeine and smoking. So you do well to avoid these food.
- Folic acid supplements are very necessary at this stage because it would help in the development of the baby's spine and brain. Take a good dosage of it.
- It is very important to start planning to eat a balanced diet especially food rich in eggs , lots of fruits, carbohydrates rich in fiber, protein and dairy foods.
- It is very necessary to take supplements rich in vitamin D, folic acid and Iron.
- You MUST avoid foods that are prone to bacteria, chemicals and/or other parasites like undercooked meat, raw eggs, mould-ripened cheeses, a meat that was cured, liver and alcohol of all types.

- As the child within you is growing teeth, so is it very necessary for you to visit a dentist especially at the seventh week of pregnancy. This is so because hormonal changes can lead to your gums being vulnerable to plaques. There's a term known as pregnancy Gingivitis or in a layman's word 'gum diseases' that occurs and this can be avoided by visiting the dentist, proper brushing and avoiding sugary snacks.

- Remember that nausea, what is commonly known as morning sickness can still occur even at the eight week of pregnancy.

- Please note that from the fourteenth week of pregnancy that it is very important to start toning your pelvic floor muscles because most times, pregnancy can put a strain on these muscles. So keeping them in good shape will save you the embarrassment that may come when you laugh out so loud.

- Avoid being stressed especially at the seventeenth week of pregnancy even when you are bursting with energy. Remember your baby needs to be cool, calm and collected.

- Whenever you feel like your emotions and

stress level are abnormal, please do not hesitate to talk to your doctor.
- At a later stage of pregnancy, say at week 21, it is normal to start feeling tired and back pains may occur. You should relax more often and try to put your feet up to calm the back pains.
- Do not forget to do some pelvic floor exercises to strengthen your pelvis. You see that at the twenty-third week of pregnancy, a simple laugh or sneeze can see a leakage or put simply see you pass urine which could be embarrassing. These exercises can avoid that.
- If you are planning to have the baby in the hospital, it would be very important to have a tour of the hospital to acquaint yourself with the facilities before the big day. This will enable ascertain whether they meet up with standards. This information will make you more comfortable and help you relax.
- With your belly-bump showing, it would be comfortable to wear loose fitting clothing.
- Keep cramps away by scratching gently or if you are a fan of yoga, you can engage yourself with it.

- With the baby bump in your sleep-way, you can try using maternity pillow which will sit between your legs supporting your bump.

- Taking your bath before going to sleep can help calm your nerves.

- At week 29, pregnancy hormones can cause digestive muscles to relax which might impact the way food digests in your stomach. So take some antacids to stop heartburn or constipation.

- From week 30, please take lots of supplements and food rich in folic acid, vitamin c and calcium.

- At a later stage of pregnancy, say at week 33, begin to engage yourself in exercises. Swimming will be a great way to exercise to give you the beautiful feeling of weightlessness.

- You may start noticing swelling of your feet. Drinking plenty of water can help reduce this swelling. It is important to note that if the swelling occurs on your face or hands, please notify your doctor or midwife, but do not panic about it, it might just be normal.

- Enjoy a foot massage at week 34 to help calm your nerve and make you relax well.

- Its very necessary to take a break from work when the pregnancy is 36 weeks old. Do not juggle work with the preparation. Stay in good shape.

- At a later stage of pregnancy, say 36 weeks, plan plenty of café dates. Any opportunity that would be make you take a walk should be welcomed.

- During pregnancy, please eat healthy snacks like oat biscuits, live yoghurts. Avoid sugary, refined and processed food.

- You don't need to increase your calories until a later stage of the pregnancy like the third trimester.

- Try to choose organic food whenever possible.

- Reduce salt and caffeinated drinks.

- It is very important to check with your doctor before taking any drugs especially pain killers.

- If you are asthmatic or diabetic, please check with your doctor before you even plan on conceiving. See your doctor immediately if it happens un-expectantly.

- For coughs and cold, try inhaling menthol and

eucalyptus.

- The best advice is to stay away from drugs during pregnancy.

- Before taking any kind of antibiotics, it is very pertinent you consul with your doctor.

- To cope with morning sickness, please endeavor to eat foods laden with vitamin B6 and zinc to help with hormonal changes in the body. Increase your intake of dairy products, leafy vegetables and lots of yeast extract. Ginger tea can also help.

- Stretch marks are sometimes inevitable. This can be controlled by a rich cream. Please speak with your beautician on these issue.

- Having sex during pregnancy will definitely not harm your baby. So enjoy the feeling and cosy up whenever you can.

# 2
# MOTHERCARE AFTER CHILDBIRTH

Mother care after childbirth starts from when the baby is born up until about six months later when the mother's body returns to its pre-pregnant state.

The basic tips to adhere to during this period include;

- A mother needs to regain her strength and that can only happen when she takes a lot of rest.
- In the first few weeks, the mother has to be relieved of all her duties so she can concentrate on baby feeding and taking care of herself.
- She has to sleep when ever the baby sleeps even if it is for a few minutes.
- The baby's crib should be close to the mother's beds o that she does not have to walk long distances to pick the baby when she cries
- Always feel free to take a nap even when there are visitors. Those few minutes can actually add up at the end of the day.
- Do some exercises like kegel exercises.

- After the first three weeks, you can have a feeding bottle where you can store up the milk at night so that someone else can feed her when she wakes at night.
- Eat a healthy diet that should contain;

    **Grains**– whole wheat, brown rice and whole meal

    **Vegetables**– legumes, peas, starchy vegetables and green vegetables.

    **Fruits**– one hundred percent fruit juice which can be canned, fresh or dried.

    **Dairy**– focus on low fat products and those that are rich in calcium.

    Protein– please eat low-fat proteinous foods, meats and poultry. Please eat more fish and, nuts, seeds and beans.
- You may need the services of a house keeper to help with laundry and doing the dishes.
- Bleeding from your uterus is common after childbirth, please use maternity pads instead of sanitary pads.
- Use nipple cream to soothe the pains and the cracking of the nipple. The pains will stop when

your body adjusts to the new life.

- To relieve breast engorgement discomforts, use warm or cold compress to your breasts.
- Eat high fiber nutrients to stimulate bowel activity and do not forget to drink plenty of water.
- As your body adjusts to childbirth, you may notice that you sweat a lot at night, please remove blankets to stay cool.

# 3
# YOUR BODY AFTER BIRTH

When you get pregnant, your body undergoes so much change both inside and outside. So this chapter discusses topics bothering on your body after childbirth. This will include stretch marks, perineal pains, skin problems, severe tear, etc.

We will also discuss and offer tips on the best methods to manage these changes.

- If you didn't have stretch marks before pregnancy, then it is very likely that your marks will fade away over time. This is caused by the stretch of your skin over your fast growing body. This marks can usually be found on the belly, bottom, thighs and breasts. Using creams will only make your body supple but will not cure the marks. Cosmetic surgery is the guarantee that you get the marks off, but they come with a price tag.

- After giving birth to your baby vaginally, it is very common for your perineum (the area between your anus and vagina) to feel very sore and painful due to the stretch of giving birth. The pains may be increased due to a tear which is usually common during vaginal child-birth. Normally, the perineum will feel so sore. To make yourself feel comfortable, lie on your tummy so the pressure is taken away from your bottom, place a cold gel pad on your perineum, have a warm bath and massage the area with hot water, wash the area with warm water to reduce stink. With time, you will get better. If the pain persists after two weeks, please consult your doctor.

- It is normal for you to bleed after child birth, this is how your body removes dirt form the lining of your womb. The bleeding could last between three weeks to six weeks. You are not required to do anything other than to use the maternity pads. If it worries you, please talk to your doctor.

- As your uterus shrinks back to its normal size, it is normal to pass blood clot. You shouldn't worry when you see those. Talk to your doctor when you think this is abnormal because sometimes a small part of the placenta may remain in the uterus causing an infection which will make you to continue passing blood clots often.

- Talk to your doctor immediately when you have the following;

- Severe and persistent headache.
- Sudden and heavy blood loss
- Increased blood pressure
- Pain in the upper part of the abdomen
- Shortness of breath
- Severe chest pain
- A severe pain in the calf
- Insomnia
- A high fever
- Difficulty in urinating after six hours of giving birth
- Unpleasant vaginal discharge
- Severe and swollen piles
- Pooing in your pants before you get to the toilet
- Constipation

- Your belly will definitely protrude after childbirth, but it would go down after some time. The degree and speed of getting back to normal depends on a number of factors. So, I urge you to be patient as your body recovers. The factors that will determine when you would recover include;

> The shape and size you were before pregnancy.
>
> How much weight you gained before you became pregnant.

The following will help you achieve results faster.

> The exercise you partake.
>
> Your genes
>
> If this is your first baby.
>
> Breastfeeding often which helps in contracting your womb.
>
> Eating healthily.

# 4

# WHEN IT IS NOT SAFE TO EXERCISE DURING PREGNANCY

Many women should be able to exercise during pregnancy but there are special conditions mainly on health grounds that should prevent the woman from any exercise.

Exercises are good because it would help you carry the weight you would gain during pregnancy and would help you sleep better. But then, it must be done with extreme care.

If she must exercise, she needs to work closely with her doctor. The following health and body conditions should prompt you to see your doctor for advice before embarking on your exercises;

- When you developed high blood pressure during pregnancy.

- When you developed pre-eclampsia during pregnancy

- When you have been told you would give birth early

- When you are carrying more than two babies in

your womb
- When your cervix is weak
- When you have irregular vaginal bleeding
- When your placenta is lying low after twenty weeks of pregnancy.
- You have an uncontrolled diabetes
- If you've had a premature baby before
- When you are a heavy smoker. You should also consider stopping the habit during pregnancy, for your safety and the safety of the child.
- When you have joint or muscle problems
- When you're over-weight.

Stop exercising when you feel any pain in your stomach or when the contractions won't go away. Stop the exercise when you feel the following;

- Dizziness
- Heart palpitation
- Pain in your back or pelvis
- Nausea or vomiting
- Sudden change in body temperature
- Swelling in your feet and hands

Seek urgent help when you experience the following;
- Leaking fluid from your vagina
- Calf pain
- Blurred vision
- Fainting feelings
- Heart beats uncontrollably fast
- Vaginal bleeding
- Your baby's movement slows down or stops.

The best exercises during pregnancy should include;
- Aerobic exercises that works your lungs and heart
- Muscle tightening exercises to increase strength and flexibility.

# 5
# HOW TO TACKLE FEVER SAFELY DURING PREGNANCY

Your temperature may rise during pregnancy, but that does not mean you should go ahead and take medications especially in the first and third trimester of pregnancy. There have been situations where people lose pregnancies due to the self-medications. So, it is very important to note this and take the right steps when you have a fever during pregnancy. Fever is not good for you or your baby.

Work with your doctor to see what works well with your system. But first, you could try taking plenty of water and rest.

Avoid taking ibuprofen during pregnany. You can take paracetamol but you must follow the dosage. In my years working in the institute of medicine, London, I have seen a case where even paracetamol caused a mis-carriage in the second month of pregnancy, so work closely with your doctor to know what works best for you.

Contact your doctor if the fever gets so high, especially when it rises beyond thirty nine degrees. They may carry out some tests if they can not easily diagnose the cause of the fever.

If your water breaks during this same period, delay not, just contact your doctor immediately.

# 6

# WHEN YOU HAVE A STILL-BORN

Losing a baby is always very devastating, but unfortunately life has to go on. In this chapter, we are going to discuss the probable causes of a still-birth and what one can do to have a healthy life after the incident.

A still birth is defined by the medical association of America as a birth of a baby who has not made any signs of life at or after twenty four weeks of pregnancy. This includes babies born at maturity which does not show any signs of life.

The causes of still-birth are so much. It includes the following;

- Placenta problems are thought to be the most common cause of still-birth. It is called placental insufficiency. This is one of the major reasons of still-birth in the world. If the placenta is not working well, it means that the blood vessels that moves blood from the mother to the child is blocked and therefore, the child may die of nutrients and oxygen lack.

- If the baby is not growing properly, that is if the baby's growth is not commensurate with the age of the pregnancy, this may lead to still-birth.

- If the mother suffers from pre-eclampsia— when the placenta is not working well— the flow of blood to the baby is disrupted which ends up killing th ebaby if the mother does not receive the treatment she deserves.
- Heavy bleeding in late pregnancy can be a cause.
- Health conditions of the mother, for instance if she has diabetes, streptococcus may also lead to still-birth.
- The age of the mother can be a factor. As women grow older, the chances of having a still-birth increases.
- Obesity, heavy drinking and smoking can also cause that.

You may want to conduct a post-mortem examination known as an autopsy to ascertain the cause of the death, but the most important thing is to go through the results if you so wish to have an autopsy. Discuss this cause(s) and find ways to avoid them if you can in the future.

People cope with the trauma of losing a child differently. The important thing here is to talk to your doctor about what to do with the breast-milk that has formed. The doctor may advise you to take some medicine to stop the production of the milk. These kinds of drugs should not be recommended if you had pre-eclampsia.

It is advisable to find a community of people who have passed through similar situations and they might be in the best position to give advice on how they managed their own situation. Exercises and talking about it in the community has been found to help a lot of women in situations like this.

The still-birth should not stop you or make you afraid of getting pregnant again. if you so wish to get pregnant again, talk to your doctor for guidance and get pregnant. If no cause was found after the autopsy, then there is no fear that should be entertained. If there was a cause, the doctor would work closely with you to avoid another incident.

# 7

# PREVENTION AND TREATMENT OF DIAPER RASH

So your baby is here, these tips will help you in taking very good care of your baby.

- Change diapers frequently most especially immediately after bowel movement.
- Endeavor to clean the area with a mild soap and water.
- Apply a diaper rash cream or commonly known as barrier cream.
- If you use cloth diapers, please always wash them in dye and detergents that has no fragrance. Always wash them in warm water. Endeavor to use bleach always because it is known to kill germs. Then double wash them in cold water to remove chemicals and soap traces.
- Don't use dryer sheets and fabric softener because they tend to contain fragrances that can

irritate your baby.

- Never use baby wipes with alcohol
- Always pat the baby's bottom with a clean towel. Though it is better to allow it to air dry since it would bring some comfort to the baby.
- don't over tighten the baby's diaper
- Always use warm water to rinse the baby's bottom as part of diaper change. This tends to suit the skin.
- Between cloth and disposable diapers, none is the best based on the fact that there is no compelling evidence, so use what works best for you and your baby.
- Before and after changing diapers, please wash your hands thoroughly to prevent the spread of bacteria and other anti-bodies.
- Applying a barrier ointment after each change prevents rashes and minimizes irritation.
- Anytime you could, please let the baby go for some hours without the diapers. It would prevent the spread of rashes.
- Mind the kind of food you eat. Certain food allergies tend to cause skin irritation on the baby. For

instance, a recent study on baby eczema has proven that eggs, peanuts, milk, wheat etc. tend to curse eczema.

- When babies tend to start eating solid food, the tendency to develop baby rash increases. Acidic foods like citrus and tomato based sauces are most likely to cause that.

- Please note that if the skin stays red between diaper changes, please use a zinc oxide diaper cream always.

- When you try to solve these problems at home and they seem to persist, please consult a pediatrician.

# 8

## DEVELOPING HEALTHY SLEEPING HABITS: BASIC DOS AND DON'TS

In this chapter, we are going to highlight the basic things to do so that you and your baby can have a good sleep at night and also teach him how to go to sleep without depending on anyone. This chapter basically solves sleep difficulties so that parents can have an uninterrupted nights' sleep.

- It is important to help your baby break away from the habit of falling asleep only with your assistance. Assistance could be nodding off in your hands and rocking, singing or nursing him in your hands. First, to break away from depending on those things, it is very important to rock the baby, but when she gets drowsy, you must put her in her crib, that way she knows how to sleep without any of your help. The last thing she sees is that she was laid to sleep alone in her crib. Comfort her in her crib, and when she cries when you are not around, you come back and soothe her, but don't remove her from crib. Repeat this often until she learns to sleep in her crib.

- Don't put the baby down with a feeding bottle. If you do that, she tends to depend on it before sleeping. She will get accustomed to sucking and will find it difficult to sleep without the dependency. Over dependency on the bottle can cause physiological problems which can interfere with her sleep.

- Decrease the amount of milk and juice given before bedtime and gradually eliminate it. The baby will soon give up the habit of her dependency on feeding before sleeping.

- Extra feeding before bedtime can stimulate the babies digestive system and cause her to wake from hunger.

- Bringing your baby to your bed will not solve any sleeping problems. Your movements alone can always wake the baby.

- When its time for the baby to start sleeping in a separate room, it is very important for you to spend some time, like ten to fifteen minutes before she sleeps so that she can identify you with the room.

# 9
# TIPS ON BABY FEEDING

Here are important tips on feeding to guide you to feed right so that your baby can have the important nutrients for general growth.

- No matter what, never give your newborn water, juice or other fluids except breast milk or formula where breastfeeding is not possible.
- Feed the newborn on demand. It is estimated that they need food every two hours on the average, that about ten to twelve times a day.
- Vitamin D is an essential vitamin in the growth of the baby. Ask your doctor on how to go about the supplement.
- When the baby closes her eyes and starts to spit out the nipple, know that the baby has had enough of the feeding. It's a sign you should stop.
- Never use food to pacify. When the baby is full, you can use other methods like rocking and singing to pacify the baby.

- The first year of the baby is largely characterized by breastfeeding, but after the first six months, you begin to put solid food in perspective so she can start learning how to eat solid food.

- While you are feeding the baby, please take note of the weight. Check with the doctor because it is expected that newborns will double their weight after the first four months and triple it after the first year. Check with the doctor so as not to exceed the guidelines.

- Gentle but consistent routines are great for better eating habits.

- When you start giving them formula, it is very important that you evaluate the formula. Just because it came out of a factory does not mean it is good to use. Be watchful for the sugar source and content. If it a corn syrup source, then it is not so great, but if it from a brown rice source, that is better. Unnecessary ingredients are not needed.

- The feeding bottle should also be checked. If it is plastic, the best are those that are BPA free. Check the label, or better yet, use glass.

- When you're feeding with bottle, please make

sure the baby is propped up at a good angle so that you don't overwhelm the baby with fluid.

- The baby might want to suck a full bottle in one gulp, so be careful with the amount she is swallowing.
- Cuddle the baby and get cozy with her. This tends to improve the bonding.
- Switch sides when feeding the baby.
- Use high quality water. Test the water for leads if you are living in an older apartment. One good trick is to allow the water flow for a while before fetching.
- Never use microwave to warm baby food.
- As she poops, please watch it and examine carefully. Watch for signs of intestinal distress, for instance a bloated belly.
- It is said that hunger is a late sign, it is very pertinent to know signs when she is hungry like licking his lips, sucking at hands, feet, tongue or clothes, turning heads frantically, mouth opening and closing e.t.c.

## DID YOUR BABY COME TOO EARLY?

Never mind if your baby was born prematurely. There

are a number of things you could do to still feed your baby properly. The thing id that your baby may not be able to take breast-milk immediately.

While the baby is getting matured, you can still save your milk in the freezer so that your baby can have it when she is ready to take milk. This will help get your milk supply established.

At first, your baby would be fed through a drip straight into her vein. This drip will contain a solution of sugar, amino acids, salts and fat. Your breast-milk could still be given to her through a pipe that would be passed through her nose into her stomach.

Once your baby is ready to have breast-milk, then this is best for her. Then you begin with the process highlighted above.

# 10

# HOW TO HOLD AND CRADLE A BABY

Knowing how to hold and cradle a baby could be a task and you must learn it to avoid causing pains on the baby. There are several different ways to hold a baby and the best choice is that which gives the baby greatest comfort and also brings comfort to the mother. The best and most common is the cradle hold which gives great support to the baby and allows for easy eye contact with the mother or the person holding them.

**THE CRADLE HOLD**

- Bend down to pick the baby. To reduce the distance that it would take to move and support the baby by the hand, it is better, safer and easier to bend towards the baby as you lift her up to your level.

- This position maximizes the amount of eye contact between the baby and the person holding her as they can only see about a foot in front of their eyes.

- Support the babies head as you lift it since they do not have the ability to that that themselves.
- Slide your stronger arm under the baby's neck and the base of the head so that your thumb supports one side of the head while the other fingers supports the other side.
- The baby's head should be cradled with the palm of your hands.
- With the other arm, place under the baby's back as if to give a hug.
- Hold the baby against your body for additional support.
- The cradle hold entails that the baby's head is resting in the bend of your elbow while your strong hand adds support from the back. Your less strong hand adds support to the baby's legs..
- The baby's head should be held higher than their feet.
- Hold the baby close to your body but it shouldn't be so tightly.
- When putting the baby down, lean over as close to the baby's crib as possible. Gently slide your arms out from under the baby and at all times,

keep supporting the baby's head.

- You can also use this cradle hold while sitting if you are afraid that you might drop the baby.
- To be more comfortable, you may consider swaddling the baby before using the cradle hold.

**TO HOLD YOUR BABY WHEN BURPING**

Choose one of these three ways;

- Sit upright. Hold your baby against your chest. As you support your baby with your shoulder, make sure your baby's chin is resting on it.
- Hold your baby across your knee, in your lap or hold her sitting up.
- When she is laying on your lap, make sure she is laying on her belly.

## 11

# THE BEST WAY TO STORE BREAST-MILK

You can store your breast-milk in a number of ways. It is very important that you keep it fresh so the baby can enjoy it.

This method is necessary if you are not taking your baby to your work place or when you are going out. It is important so that your baby can continue to get the nutritional benefits of breast-milk. This will also keep your milk supply flowing.

The tips include;

- Keep it at room temperature of 25 degrees Celsius and no more than six hours.

- In a cool box with ice packs or blocks for up to twenty hours.

- In a refrigerator at 4 degrees Celsius or colder and for up to five days. Store it away from meat and other uncooked foods. This is to avoid being contaminated with the smell of those of foods.

- In the compartment of a freezer for up to two weeks.
- You can add new breast-milk to the one in the freezer so long as it was stored or milk on the same day.
- Always sterilize your containers so your baby can always get good quality and healthy breast-milk.
- Wash your hands thoroughly before milking your breast and keep everything as clean as possible.
- Lest you forget, always label your containers with the right dates so that you don't get confused .
- Use the first in, first out method.
- Your breast nozzle should always be kept clean.
- You can freeze your milk, but when doing so, keep a little space or a gap at the top of the container. It is common for the breast milk to expand and occupy space when frozen.
- Please never use microwave to defrost your frozen breast-milk, if you do that, it is no longer breast milk. Always defrost it under normal cold temperature.

## 12

# HOW AND WHEN TO INTRODUCE SOLID FOOD

Experts suggests that you start giving your baby solid food from when he is six months old. When you start, you may want to start with well mashed foods like cooked potatoes and pureed fruits like banana and mango. Cereals such as rice, maize and cornmeal can also be used.

The tips include the following;

- Depending on what works for you, you can introduce solid food to your baby before, during or after breast-milk. Test to know how hot the food is by placing little at the back of your wrists before giving it to the baby.

- Be patient with your baby as they learn these new flavours because it might take them a while to get used to them.

- It may take them time to learn how to swallow, chew and the motion of grinding. Add less and less liquid making the food texture thicker until the baby adapts to the new form of food.

- When they get used to cereals, vegetables and fruits, gradually add other food types and increase the number of times he eats the solid food. When he is seven months, you make the baby eat solid food three times.

- Make sure that the food is balanced and contains all the essential nutrients. For instance, a typical day may contain a combination of breast milk or formula milk, iron fortified cereal, vegetables, small amounts of meat, poultry, fish, yoghurt and fruits.

- Don't you ever give your baby a mould-ripened food or soft cheeses.

- By now you should know when your baby is full. When he begins to play with the food or closes his mouth, he's probably had enough.

- Sometimes, you may allow your baby to feed themselves when they are up to age. This is called baby-led weaning.

# 13
# WHAT TO DO WHEN YOUR BABY CHOKES

Accidents do happen. Many accidents are nothing to worry about. It is good to know what to do in the event of any accident. These helpful tips will help you know exactly what to do when your child chokes on an object.

- If your child is choking and by chance you do not know the object, please never put your fingers in her mouth as you stand the risk of pushing the object further down his throat.

- If he is unable to breathe, cough or cry, try to dislodge the object by blowing the back with your flats of your hand or thrust his chest.

- Hold the child underneath your arm holding him upside down, deliver the thrusts or the blows.

- Check the mouth after this if the object is not dislodged. If there is an object, use your fingers to remove the object.

- If after three trials and the object is still not dislodged, then it is probably time to call the ambulance. Continue with the process of trying to dislodge the object until the ambulance arrives.

## 14

# IF YOUR CHILD BEGINS TO VOMIT

It is important to know what's normal and what abnormal when it comes to your baby's vomiting. Anything can cause a baby to vomit. It could be car sickness, indigestion, a prolonged bout of crying or coughing. So it is normal to see a lot of vomiting in your baby's first few years.

- An attack of vomiting should subside after 6 to 24 hours after it starts. You shouldn't worry about the treatment apart from giving him plenty of water to prevent dehydration. As long as the baby looks healthy and continues to gain weight.

- Apart from the above, when the baby's vomiting is accompanied with diarrhea, then it seems the baby has a tummy infection, an ear infection, a cold and a urine infection.

- Call your doctor when you notice any of the following:

- Dehydration which may come with dry mouths, lack of tears and a dry or fewer wet diapers.

When the vomiting is accompanied with fever, not breast-feeding, severe irritability, a swollen abdomen, persistent forceful vomiting, blood or vile in the vomit and vomiting with a great force.

- If your baby attends crèche, keep him at home for at least 48 hours after the last vomit to monitor.
- Never give your baby anti-nausea medicines unless they are prescribed by the doctor.
- Keep your baby hydrated when he begins to vomit.
- After a period of 12 hours after his last vomit, you can begin to give him his normal diet while continuing to monitor him.
- Help him rest as sleep can help settle him to relieve his need to vomit.

# 15

# HOW TO EASE THE DISTRESS OF TEETHING

Teething can be a lot of pain to the baby. The reasons for the pains comes from the teeth pushing through the gums. If the under-listed signs worry you, please do not hesitate to see the doctor. The length of time depends on the baby's body. It could start at six months up until the baby's first birthday.

The signs include the following:

- Sleeplessness at night and refuses to sleep during the day. This is not the only sign, so its necessary to check for other signs.

- Red and swollen gums

- Flushed cheeks apparently from the pains

- Gum rubbing and/or sucking

- Always irritable and unstable

- May develop high temperature and diarrhea

- Finally, not feeding well

**The best ways to soothe the pains include:**

There are plenty of things you could do to reduce the pains of your baby during the teething period. These may include one or more of the following:

- You could rub a clean finger over the baby's sore gum to numb the pains. But note that this has a temporal effect.
- You can try giving the baby a teething ring. It has been proven that a solid silicone based teething ring is a lot better than other types.
- You may want to give your baby something to chew at. Something like a dummy which will help in soothing the pains. Cool soft foods can also work, like banana.
- Many times, the baby just needs a cuddle when every other thing fails.
- Teething gels can also work based on the report we receive from mothers. If you opt for this, please use one that is sugar free.
- You can also give her infant paracetamol

# 16

# HOW TO HANDLE YOUR BABY'S HICCUPS

Hiccups are very common with baby's under a year old. They easily get a hiccup after a meal, it probably should be a hiccup that shouldn't bother him so much. It is usually referred to as posseting or reflux. This is normal as long as the baby is feeling well. Just make sure you have a tissue or muslin around to clean the mess.

You may also want to try this:

- Feed your baby in an upright position
- After each feed, hold the baby in an upright position for up to twenty minutes
- Try giving your baby smaller but more frequent feeds so that the system can mature gradually to take in more food
- Burp the baby every two or three minutes when feeding him with feeding bottles.
- If the hiccups becomes severe, please talk to your doctor.

# 17
# WHEN IT IS IMPORTANT TO SEE THE DOCTOR.

You know since your baby's immune system is still developing, it is very important that you prepare your mind because they will be more prone to mild sicknesses than older kids. Err on the side of caution and see your doctor even when your instincts say all is right. There is nothing to be scared of because once they get the right treatment, they recover faster.

The symptoms that should make you see the doctor ASAP include:

- When the diarrhea persists for more than 12 hours.
- Repeated vomiting and most importantly, if the vomiting comes with rash, fever or diarrhea.
- When she has a fever that is more than 38 degrees Celsius and she is still under three months old.
- If the fever is 39 degrees Celsius and she is older than three months old.
- If an object is lodged into her ear, nose, mouth or

vagina. Be careful while trying to remove it but on the other hand, call the doctor too.

- A bum especially if it comes with a blister.
- If she cries persistently beyond what is acceptably normal.
- A vomit that is accompanied with blood.
- A barking cough especially when it is accompanied with a wheezing sound.
- A rash that cannot be explained.
- Dehydration (dry lips)and has refused to take water or any drink.
- If she has watery and/or pinky eyes with other symptoms like dark yellow urine and fewer wet diapers.
- If she becomes unusually irritable and moody.
- If there is any discharge from the ears , eyes or genitals.
- Call emergency number 999 when the baby is unconscious, shows signs of meningitis (a fever with cold hands, pale blotchy skin, a purple red rash, unusual crying or moaning etc.), has a seizure, becomes unwell after swallowing something harmful or poisonous and she is breathing

abnormally.

- If she has a cut that keeps bleeding profusely.
- Has a serious fall
- Gets a serious bump on the head.
- Has a severe stomach pain
- Swallows anything that may be poisonous.

REFERENCES

www.babycentre.co.uk

# 18
# DEALING WITH ALLERGIES AS IT AFFECTS YOUR BABY

An allergy can be simply be describes as when your child's immune system reacts to something that is usually harmless. The substance or food is known as an allergen.

The body's immune system sees the allergen as an attacker and promptly reacts to this allergen by producing anti-bodies. This continues to happen when the baby's body meets with the substance.

Allergies are hereditary and can be out-grown especially if the child's allergen is milk which is the most common cause of allergies in children. But scientific reports has it that children who are allergic to milk may later develop asthma or hay fever in the future.

Allergies can only be diagnosed through an allergy test

The symptoms of an allergy includes, but not limited to these because allergies are not easy to detect because these symptoms can be caused by other sicknesses.

- Watery, itchy eyes and nose
- Skin rash
- Swollen lips and mouth
- Itchy mouth
- Vomiting
- Diarrhea
- Wheezing in severe cases
- Throat and tongue swelling

Medications can't cure an allergy. So its better you take the child to see an allergy doctor who would most probably perform an allergy test on the child.

If your child is allergic to dusts, then you have to do a lot of cleanings to reduce the amount of dusts in the room.

If he is allergic to pets, then you might as well limit the pets to one room and make them spend more time outside of the house.

If the allergy is caused by any kind of food, replace them with other kinds of foods.

# 19
# HOW TO BATH YOUR BABY SAFELY

Follow these rules to make bath fun as well as safe.

- Make sure the water has the right temperature. You might want to test the warmth of the water by using a thermometer. The water must be warm but not hot and mix it well
- The water should feel neither hot nor cold.
- The depth of the water should be about 13cm deep, enough so that the baby's shoulders are submerged in the bath. This is very essential if the baby is between new and six months old.
- For older babies, never fill the bath more than the baby's waist.
- When you lower your baby into the bath, make sure you support him from behind– under of her neck and shoulders, then use another hand to wash him. Keep a firm hold on your baby and support her head above the water.
- Never leave your baby alone in the bath. In a sur-

vey, a baby every year drowns in the bath due to negligence. So always stay close to your baby.

- Note that babies can easily down even in a bath that is 3cm deep if left alone.
- You can bath your baby between two to three times a day.
- Choose a mild liquid soap and cleanser to maintain the baby's natural skin barrier.
- When the baby is some months old, you may want to incorporate the bath as night time routine so that the baby can get used to it.
- To solve dry or irritated skin if your baby has one, add a little bath emollient to the water.
- Once your baby is up to two months old, you can take a bath with your baby but you need to be careful. You will need someone to hand over the baby to you and take it from you when you are through so you can get out of the bath.
- Make sure everything you need in the bath is close-by.
- It is so important we say this again, never leave your baby alone in the bath. If you must answer the door or the phone, take your baby with you.

# 20

# DOES YOUR BABY HAVE ECZEMA?

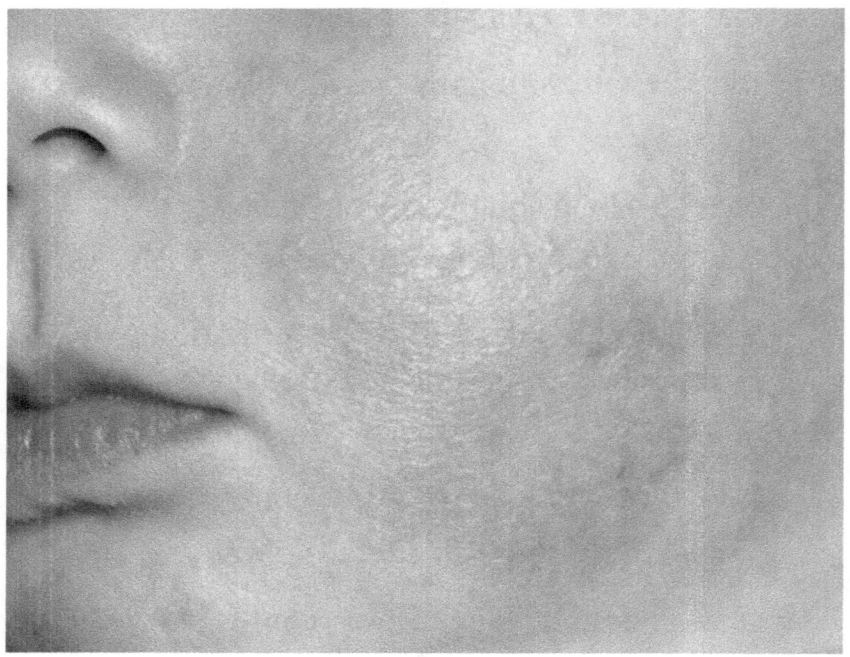

Eczema is a skin disease that is usually characterized by dryness and itching on the skin. It is common with children. It affects about a fifth of children. It usually appears on your child before they become two years.

Eczema can't be cured but it can be controlled with the right treatments. Most children out grow them in their teens.

It is mostly inherited. Eczema means that your baby's skin barrier doesn't work so well which makes it drier. This will make the skin open to infections and allergens.

The causes of eczema is not well documented. The scientific reports says that the study is on-going but they went on to say that genes play a major role in the cause of it.

In the treatment of eczema, use a ointment known as nixoderm which is rubbed in the area affected, this will keep the area moisturized as it controls the eczema.

You can use emollient cream with a short course of steroids if the eczema is mild. Steroid creams are safe if used correctly. Please work with your doctor on this.

If the eczema is itchy and stopping the baby from sleeping, you may use oral antihistamines.

If the eczema is strong, you may use stronger steroid creams.

Other treatments may use bandages and wet wrapping, where they are soaked in emollient creams and other ointments.

Breast-feeding exclusively may prevent eczema. If the eczema becomes infected, then you will need antibiotics to treat the infection. You can tell if they are infected when the skin becomes broken and emitting fluids due to severe itching.

**ADD THIS TO THE TREATMENT:**

Other self-help tips include;

- Make a record of what triggers eczema on your baby's skin then discuss it with your doctor.

- Experts say certain kinds of food can cause eczema, but do not change your baby's food without discussing with your doctor.

- Keep your house clean as dusts can also cause eczema as revealed by a recent study.

- Cotton clothing may help because clothes that make your baby too warm may worsen eczema

- Keep her nails short so that she does not use it to scratch up the skin.

# 21

# WHEN YOUR BABY CRIES TOO MUCH (COLIC)

Colic refers to when your baby's cries total over three hours in any given day, then there is something wrong, but you need not worry over it. Colic will never hurt your baby. Stay as calm as possible. You can talk to the doctor or to other moms who have had the same experience in your community. You can also know if the baby has colic if she cries becomes frequent, intense and inconsolable. Another way is when she cries and arches her back or she pulls her legs to her tummy.

However, excessive crying can be upsetting and can even make you cry, here are some things you can do to soothe her, because there are times your baby cries for no just reason. Take these soothing tips:

- Massage her tummy in a clockwise movement to remove trapped air and poo.
- Use a dummy for him to suck.
- Burp the child after every meal, this makes them comfortable.

- Try anti-gas remedies. This means that you have to make sure that she is not sucking air while sucking from the bottle.
- Bring her close to your heart so she could hear your heart-beat. This may cool her down and stop her from crying.
- Swaddle him if she is less than a month.
- Dim the lights and make the room quiet around her.
- Take her for a ride in her toy car.
- A warm bath may be of help.
- Rock her and see if she might sleep.

**WHY YOU HAVE TO SEE THE DOCTOR ABOUT COLIC**

See your doctor immediately if the colic comes with the following;

- If the cry is high-pitched
- If she vomits a greenish fluid
- Has blood in her poo
- Has fewer wet nappies or has a dry mouth
- Takes less water or other fluids

## 22
# YOUR BABY HAS COLD SORES

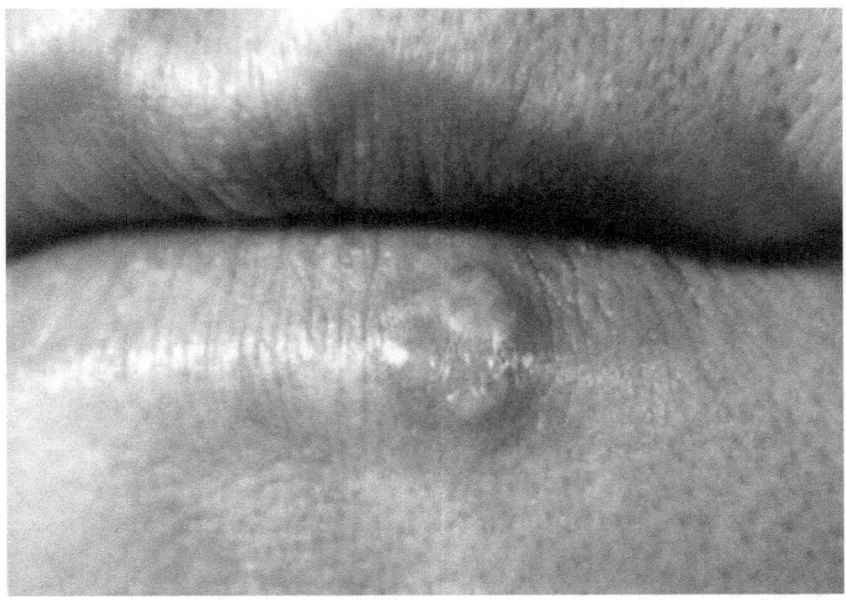

Cold sores usually appear as clusters of tiny blisters on the lip. The babies feel a tingling, itching, burning, numbness or pain on the lip or mouth area which makes them to cry so often. It can also appear on the insides of his mouth, on the roof or his gum.

They are caused by the herpes simplex virus type 1. it is very contagious and its very likely that someone with a cold sore had kissed your baby. The person may not have a visible sore but may carry the virus in their saliva.

Do not hesitate to call the doctor right away when you suspect your baby has a cold sore. It may take some time before it manifests on his body due to the baby's immunity he received from you in the Uterus.

The early symptoms include;

- Swollen gums
- A sore mouth
- Fever
- Swollen lymph glands in his neck
- A cluster of small blisters near his lips

The best way to prevent your baby from cold sores is to identify and prevent him from meeting those with cold sores. That also includes you. You should not kiss your baby if you have a cold sore.

Try to prevent your baby from any factor that triggers cold sores like exposing him to sunlight. On any sunny day, please cover your baby with a sunscreen. You can also apply a lip balm that contains a sunscreen.

Ordinarily, the cold sores will just go away on its own, but in the mean time, there are things you can do to make him feel better;

- You can get some OTC drugs and apply on the baby. You can ask your doctor for the best.
- You can apply ice to the sore to ease the pain. A single dose of children paracetamol can also ease the pains.
- Stop the baby from touching his eyes and the areas surrounding the cold sore. This will stop the transfer of the cold sore to his eyes.
- Keep him neat and clean to stop him from transferring the cold sores to other parts of the body.
- If he is too weak to feed, please make sure he is not dehydrated. Always get him extra water.

# 23
# IMMUNIZING YOUR BABY

This chapter will show you how to create a chart so that you know when to immunize your baby. It would show you when and what to expect.

**2 months old**

When your baby is two months old, you take the baby for a single injection that would prevent him from having Diphtheria, whooping cough, tetanus, polio, influenza type B and hepatitis B.

Another PCV injection will be given to prevent pneumococcal infection.

Another will be given to prevent meningitis B.

Finally, one oral does would be given to prevent Rotavirus.

**1 year old**

At one year, the baby would be immunized against haemophilus influenza type B and meningitis C. one injection would take care of that.

Another injection will take care of measles, mumps

and rubella.

One injection each will take care of meningitis B and Pneumococcal infection.

**2 years old**

One nasal spray of live attenuated influenza vaccine to take care of flu.

**3 years old.**

One nasal spray of live attenuated influenza vaccine to take care of flu.

**3 years and 4 months**

One injection of Dtap/IPV to take care of Diptheria, tetanus, whooping cough and polio.

Another injection to tackle measles, mumps and rubella.

**4 years to 8 years (Every September)**

One nasal spray to combat flu. The baby would be sprayed with a live attenuated influenza vaccine.

## 24

# TREATING INSECT BITES

There is nothing to worry about insect bites. These stings may give your baby a fright and will cause him a lot of pain and itching. The area may become swollen and a red mark may appear. The mark may be accompanied by a lump. The lump will definitely disappear after a few hours, but wouldn't stay for up to a day. This description is typically of a mosquito, midge or a flea bite and you really have nothing to worry about.

If your baby is stung by a bee, try removing the sting with the sharp edge of your finger nails, and be careful not to push more of the venom in to your baby's body. Then wash the area with soap and plenty of water.

THEN DO THE FOLLOWING;

- You can apply an ice pack or anything cold to the swelling to reduce the itching and the swelling.

- Stop the baby from scratching the area of the bite. Keep his fingernails short at all times, because this alone will save other problems and also stop him from scratching.

- You can use certain creams to combat the itching like corticosteroid cream but do not apply it to the skin if your baby's skin is broken.
- If the pain is so intense, you can give the baby infant paracetamol or ibuprofen.
- Check to know if the bite is infected. You can do this by checking if the bite area has a firm bump, a permamnent swelling, a sore and red streaks. If any of these is present, then the baby is infected. Also if the baby scratches too much, it is also a sign that the bite is infected.
- Take the baby to the doctor if you have any signs of infections from the bite.
- If the bite leads to an allergy which has the following symptoms– vomiting, swelling in the face, diarrhea, dizziness, a rapid pulse and breathing problems. This allergy could be life threatening, so you need to see a doctor immediately.
- When you are going on a journey, always protect your baby from insect bites and stay away from areas where there are bees and warps.

IF THE BITE COMES FROM A TICK

A tick is a wingless insect which usually attaches itself to the skin of animals to feed on their blood. They can also live on humans. It would take some time before you know your baby has a tick. As it feeds, a swelling which may be up to 1cm long will form and it would be easier to see.

If you notice a tick, remove it as soon as possible. Use fine and neat tweezers to remove it. Use the tweezers to grab the tick. Gently pull straight up until all parts of the tick is removed. Please never twist the tick as you are removing it to avoid it breaking off. Wash your hands with clean water and soap after removing it then dress the tick bite with an antiseptic and plenty of water.

# 25

# TREATMENT OF SKIN RASHES

There are many benign spots, blemishes and birthmarks that can be found on the skin of the baby. There are some that you need to worry about. For instance, milia and spots are completely harmless.

There are some that will give you something to worry about. This section will treat as many body rashes as possible so that you know what to do when you find it.

BABY ACNE, MILIA AND SPOTS

Some babies have a few red spots over their noses

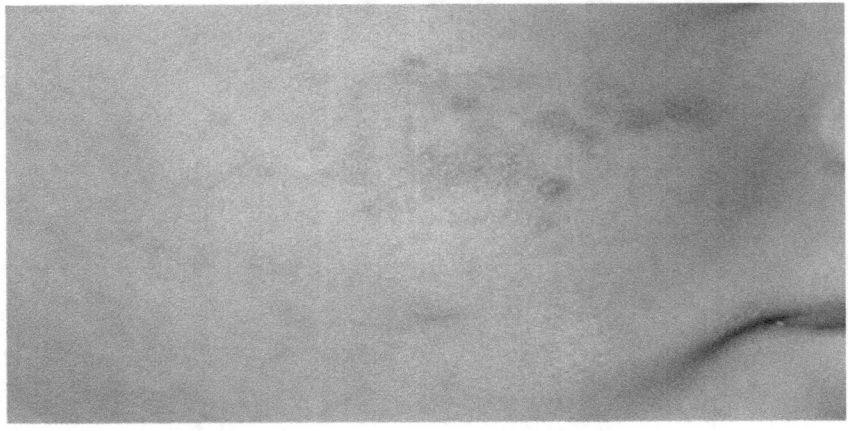

and cheeks and there is no cause for alarm because it usually clears off by itself within six weeks. Never try to remove the acne by yourself. It does not bother the baby. Just clean the baby's body as this will clear away.

BLEPHARITIS/STYES/CHALAZION

A stye is a boil at the base of an eyelash. This begins with a red bump that appears at the edge of his eyelid. It would get larger and burst after a few days.

Blepharitis is a bacterial infection that causes the eyelash follicles at the base of the eyelid to become inflamed. Do not worry about it because it would not damage your child's eye.

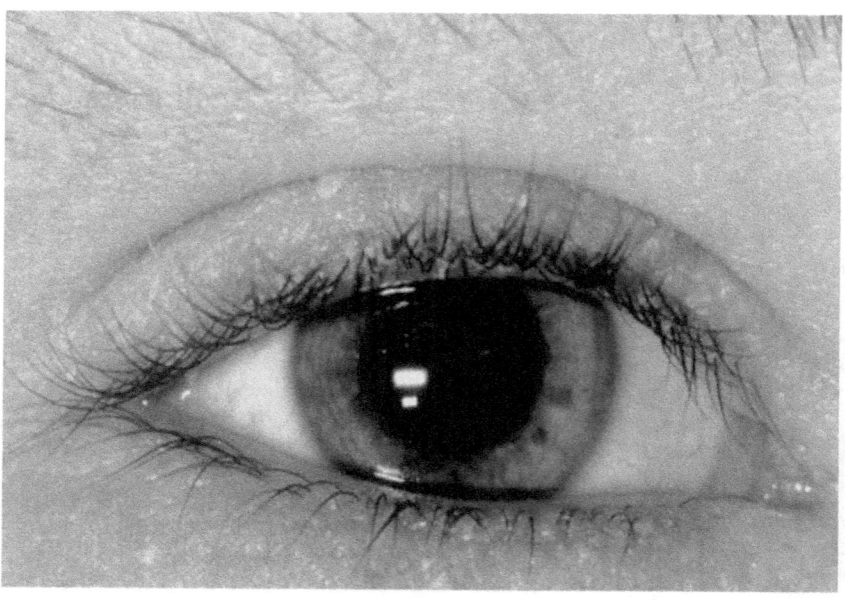

Blepharitis can be treated by a doctor who is likely to

prescribe a routine cleaning of the eye and improved eye hygiene.

If it looks like your baby has a bump under his eyelids, he may have a chalazion and its usually painless. If your baby still has a chalazion after a month, see your doctor.

CHICKEN POX

This does not need any introduction. The symptoms includes fever, nausea, headache, muscle aches and loss of appetite.

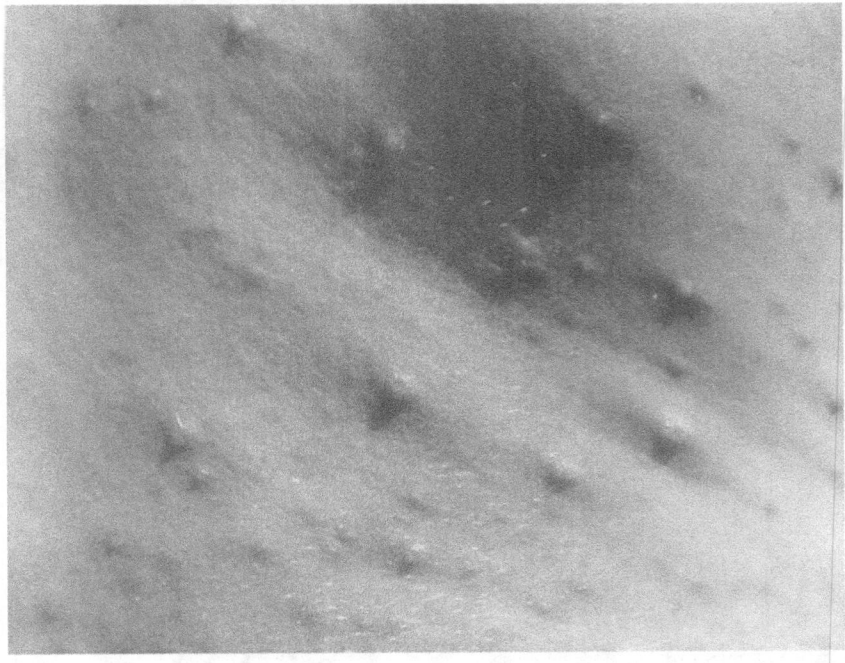

Take your baby to see the doctor if you think the baby

has chicken pox because chicken pox can be very dangerous and can cause other complications. You can help relieve the baby's conditions with infant paracetamol and also rubbing calamine lotion on his body. Give plenty of water to prevent dehydration.

Note that if you have never had chicken pox before, then it is possible for you to contact it because it is very contagious, but at all times, protect yourself to avoid shingles, which is another form of the virus that causes chicken pox. Keep the baby away from pregnant women who have not had chicken pox before.

CRADLE CAP

This is a rare skin condition which resembles a dandruff and can show up a red patch on your baby's

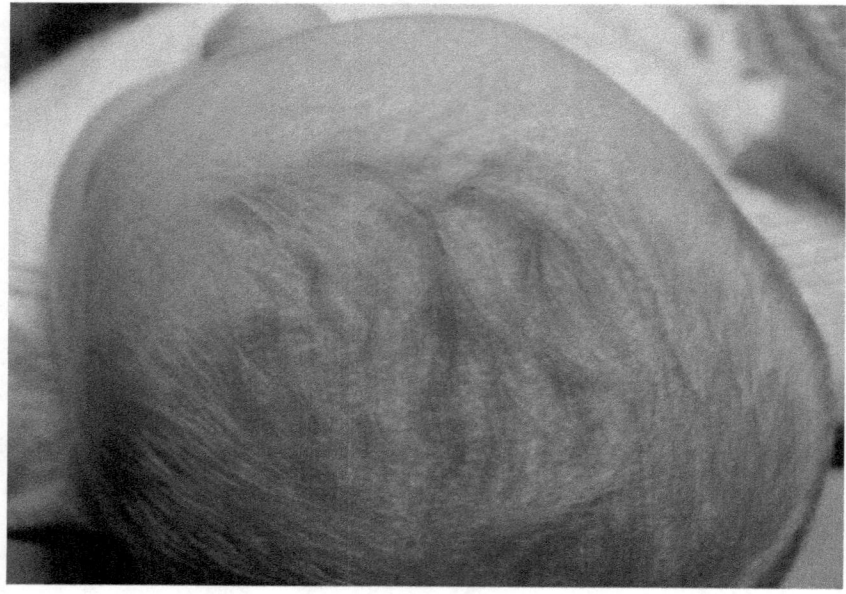

scalp, covered with greasy, yellow scaly patches. They can become flak and fall off just like dandruff, but it may come off with your baby's hair. It can take up the entire scalp and can even extend to the shoulders, neck, face, armpits, nose and nappy area.

To treat this, wash your baby's hair regularly with shampoo and then loosen the flakes using a soft brush. Rub a mild baby oil on the affected area. If this continues over time, please see a doctor.

## FOLLICULITIS

If your baby has pustules around some of his hair follicles, it is very likely that he has folliculitis. This usually appear in crops, and it may appear on your baby's neck, arms, legs, armpits and bottom. If you suspect your baby has this, please see a doctor immediately.

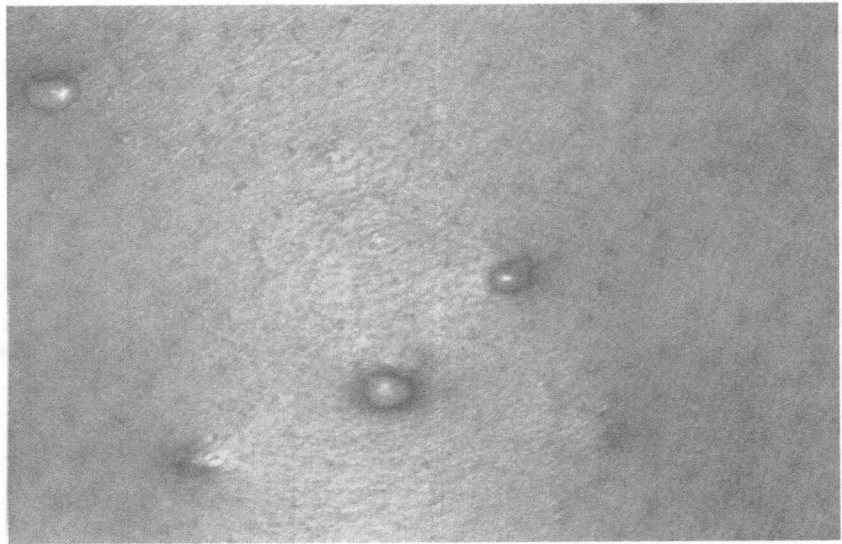

## HIVES

Hives is characterized by small raised patches known as wheals that appears suddenly. These wheals can be red or white and can be itchy. These wheals can join together which might it look so extensive. Hives may develop by allergies from certain kinds of food like nuts, cow's milk and some kinds of medicine like anti-inflammatory drugs like ibuprofen. If you suspect that

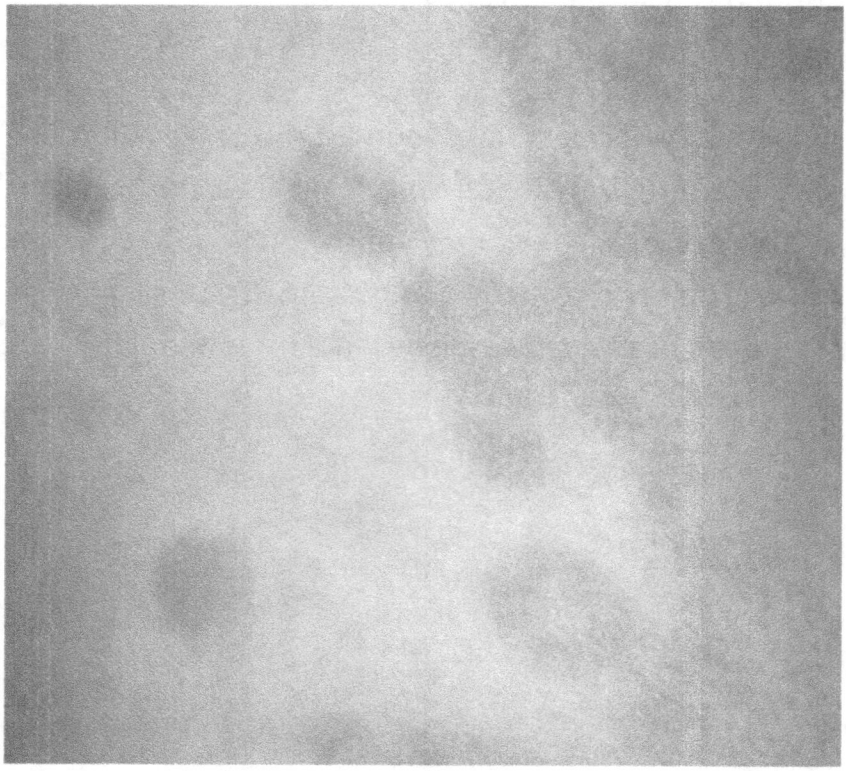

the hives are caused by any allergic reaction, please see the doctor immediately because it could be signs of Anaphylaxis. Watch out for wheezing, difficulty in breathing, loss of consciousness, skin that feels cold and clammy, nausea, vomiting and a rapid heart rate.

In treating hives, the condition may disappear on its own, but if the hives become swollen and itchy, take the baby to see the doctor. You can do the following at home to bring relief to the baby;

- Use calamine lotion
- Use clothes made with natural fibres, like cotton.
- Keep his nails short
- Watch out for detergents which may make the condition worse.

## IMPETIGO

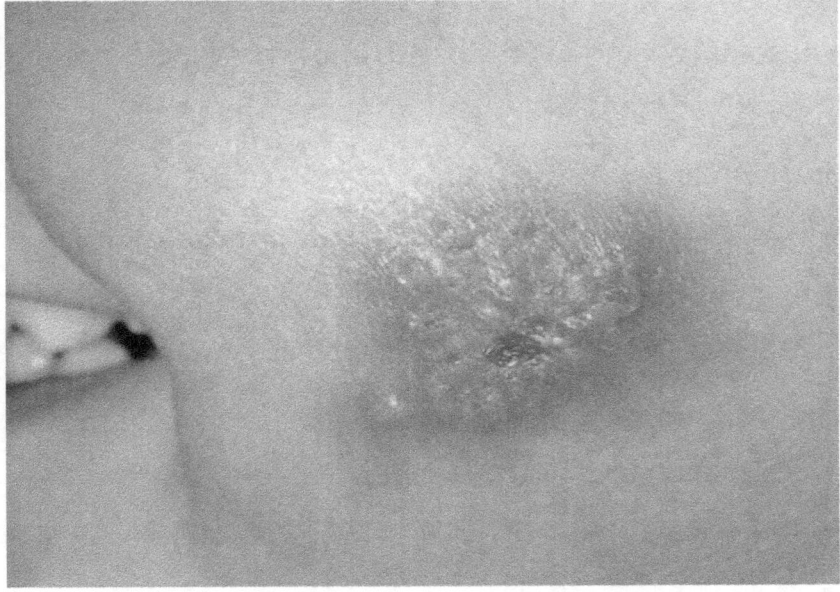

Just like the picture above, impetigo is usually a cluster of blisters which begins around the cheek, nose and mouth and can spread to other parts of the body, and usually not painful, but can be itchy. They can enter the baby's body through cold sores.

Take the baby to see the doctor if you suspect that she has impetigo. The doctor would prescribe an antibiotic cream that you can use to rub on the area. It is also very important to keep the area clean. Wash your hands before and after applying the cream or use gloves, trim the baby's fingernails and dress him in loose cotton clothes.

Take the baby to see the doctor if the home treatment seems not to be working or the fever is not subsiding. A skin sample would be taken to determine the cause of the impetigo, so as to know the kind of treatment to administer.

JAUNDICE

This is a condition where the babies liver which is too small to process the extra bilirubin which is produced by the red blood cells metamorphosis.

This is how you test if your baby has jaundice in the first few hours of birth. In a well-lit room, gently press your fingers on the baby's nose or forehead. As you

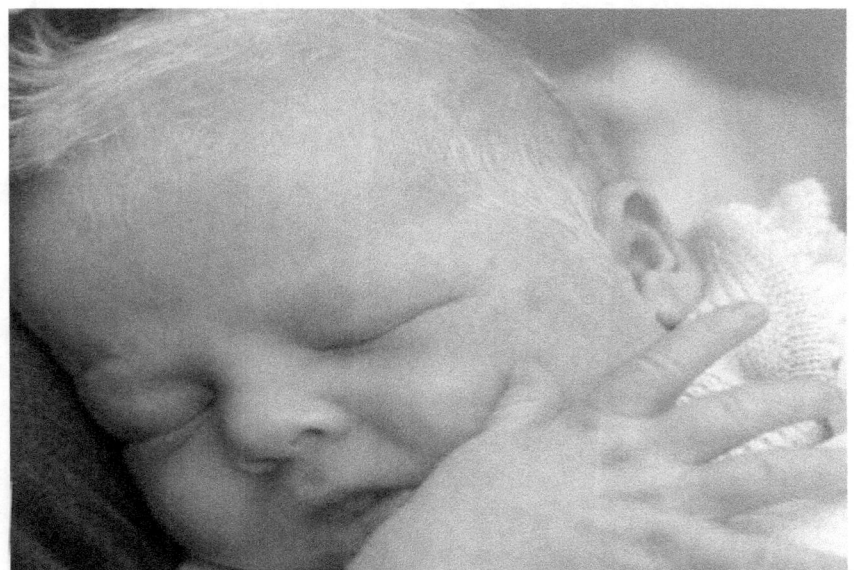

release your finger and there's a yellow tinge to her skin, then there is need to talk to your doctor or midwife incase your baby needs treatment to clear the jaundice.

Please do this test in the first twenty four hours after birth. When your test is positive in the first twenty four hours, please see a doctor immediately because the jaundice could rise to a dangerous level.

MENINGITIS

This is a very serious condition that is not easily detected. You can detect it when you place a glass against the rash and it does not disappear. The problem is that the rash does not appear until the disease is at an advance stage.

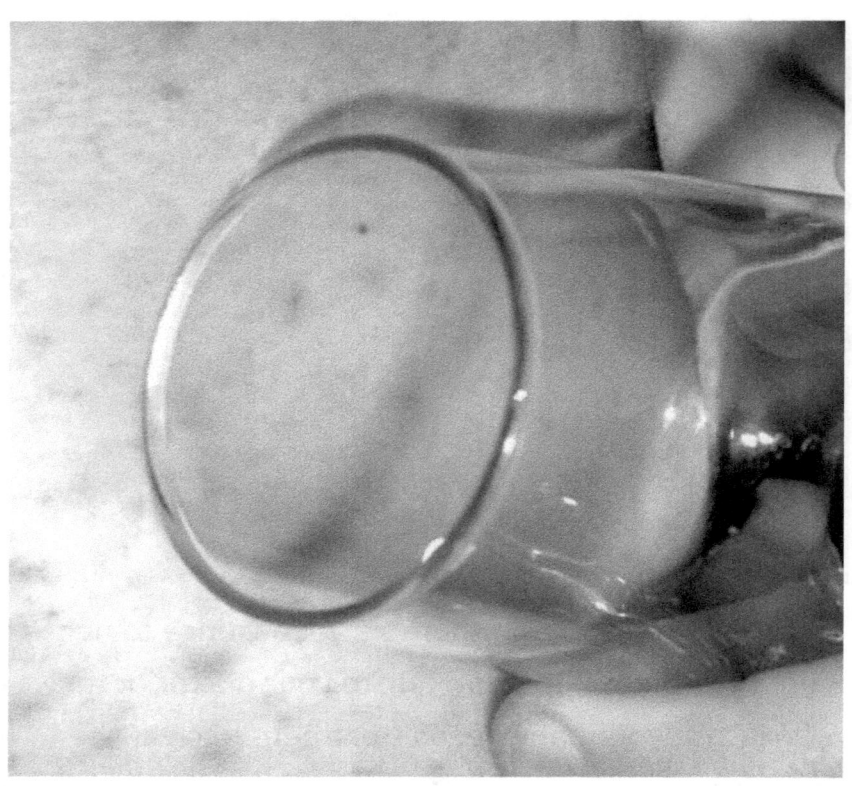

Early symptoms include;

- Pale or blotchy skin
- Vomiting and refusing food
- Refuses to be touched
- A bulging fontanelle (the soft spot on your baby's head)
- When he gives a shrill cry
- Drowsy and floppy

## NAPPY RASH

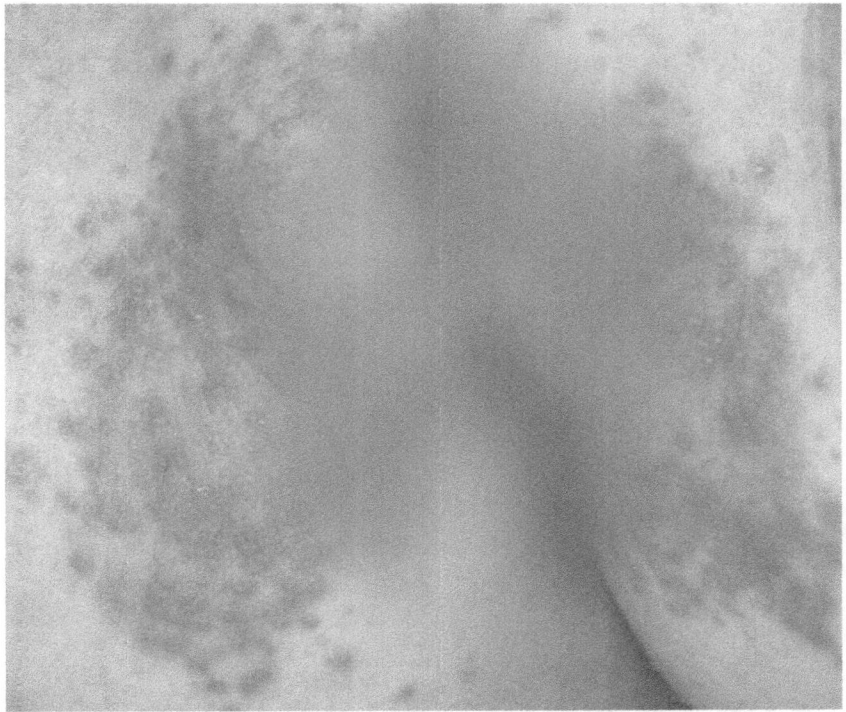

Your baby may develop nappy rash which is mainly caused by wetness. It has other causes which may include allergies. This rash covers the places that always covered with napkin-buttocks, genitals and the folds of her thighs.

You can prevent this rash by changing your baby's napkin regularly, clean thoroughly and apply barrier cream. Do not use talcum powder because it may end up irritating the skin.

Get the doctor if the rash gets worse.

In treating the rash, change the nappy as often as possible, keep the affected areas as clean as possible, use barrier creams and give the baby as many nappy free times as possible.

RINGWORM

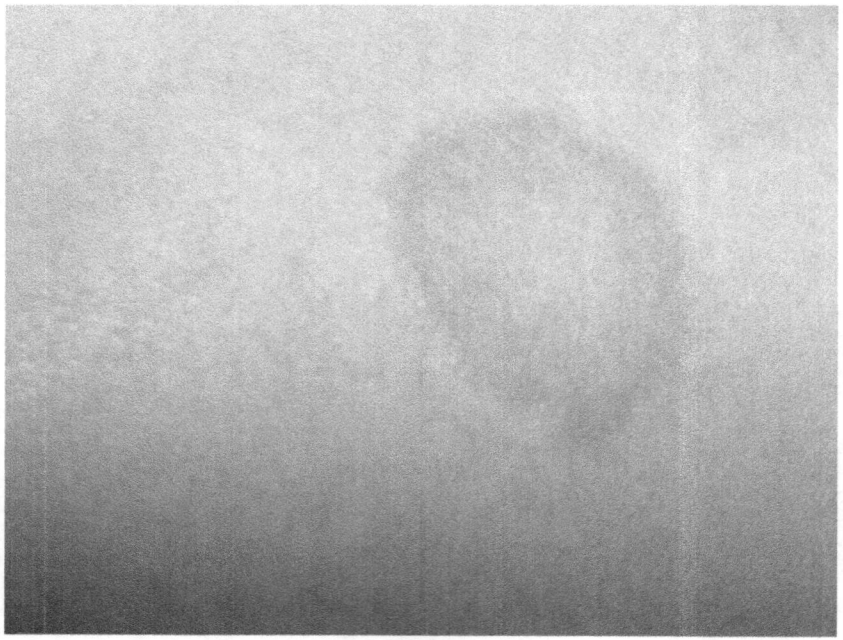

Ringworms are caused by fungus on the skin of the baby and can be itchy. As the fungus grows, it becomes larger and raging in size. This rash are red-like rings and can happen on any part of the body. It is usually dry and crusty on the scalp.

It usually enters the body through a broken part of the skin, a cut or scratch. It is usually transferable when the baby comes in contact with something a carrier uses like the comb.

It is easily treatable with an OTC antifungal cream, but first, you must identify the right cream by using a small amount of the cream first to watch if it is good enough for your baby.

Rub the cream in the affected area and extend a little above the area to stop the spread.. Improve hygiene around your baby. Keep his fingers short to stop the baby from spreading the infection on his body. Watch the baby closely and advice family members with ringworms not to come close to the baby to stop the baby from contacting the infection.

SCABIES

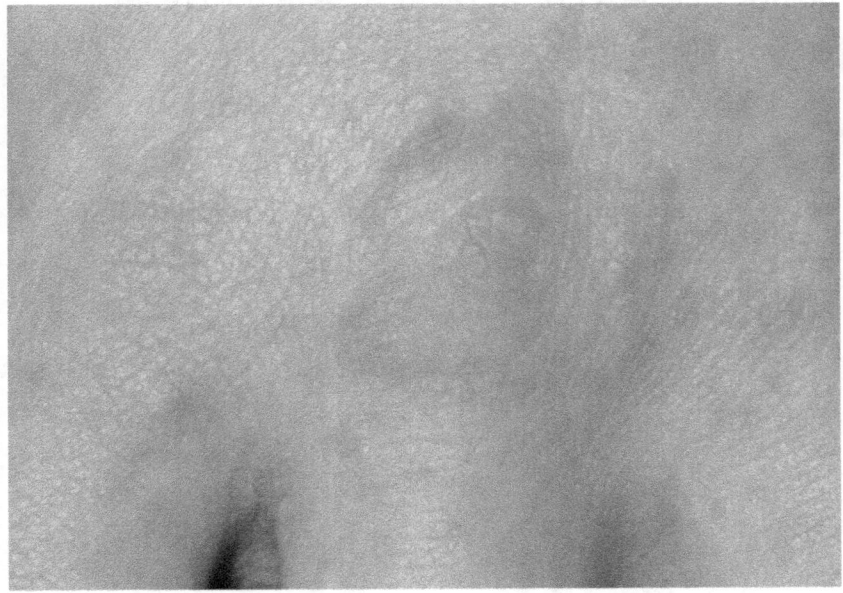

Scabies is an irritation on the skin of babies which is caused by mite parasites living and burrowing under the skin. The rash which is usually bumpy are as a result the saliva, eggs and excretes of the mites. Scabies generally is not harmful but can bring a lot of discomfort to the babies by way of itch. It is contacted through skin contact of someone who has it.

Scabies is largely characterized by large red scattered bumps usually between the babies fingers, his wrists, his armpits and on the outside of his elbows. It may also spread to the belly, scalp, the palms of his hands and on the sides and soles of his feet.

You should take the baby to see the doctor to conduct a test. If is confirmed that the baby has scabies, the doctor will prescribe a cream. Spread the cream around his body from the neck down. The cream will work best when applied on a dry, cool body. Protect your baby from sucking the cream from his fingers by covering the finger he sucks often with socks. Be patient with the treatment because it could take as much as three weeks before the itching stops.

You can go ahead and treat the rest of the family with the same cream to avoid a re-occurrence.

## SLAPPED CHEEK

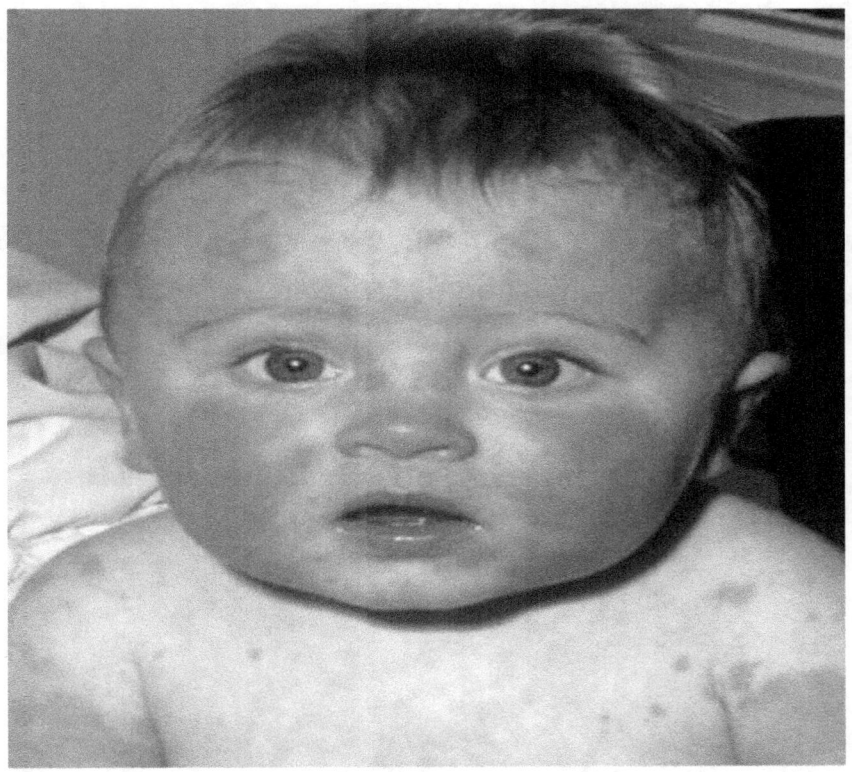

If your baby has a blotchy red rash on his cheek which may also appear on his limbs and body, then it is possible he has developed a slapped cheek syndrome which is caused by a virus.

Since it's a virus, a slapped cheek should be allowed to run its course and within the period, and after it would just go away. In the meantime, you can do certain things to bring comfort to the baby.

- Plenty of rest
- Encourage him to take extra breast or formula feed.
- Infant paracetamol can help with the pains.

Slapped cheek syndrome is generally a mild sickness but it can be very dangerous for babies with sickle cell.

TONSILLITIS

The tonsils is an almond-shape organ in the mouth

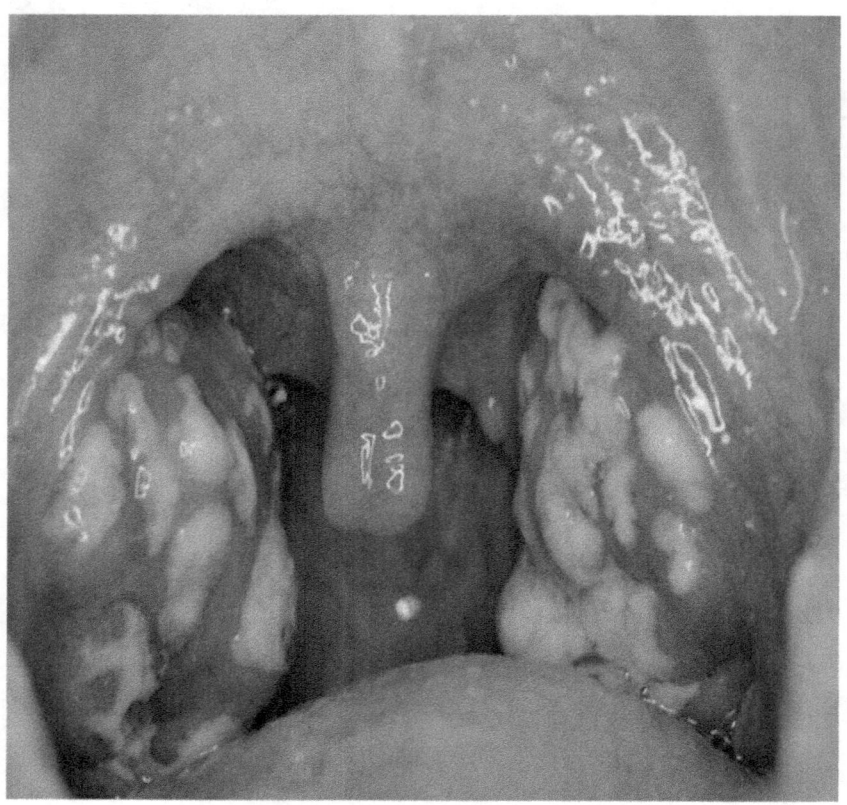

that filters parasites out of the throat, but when the become infected, it can cause the tonsils to swell and become inflamed.

The symptoms are that;

- Your baby has difficulty swallowing food.
- Refuses to eat
- Fever
- Sore throat
- Swollen glands in the neck and jaw
- Breathing through the mouth while sleeping
- Difficulty is speaking
- Headache
- In severe cases, white spots will appear on the tonsils.

Most cases of this ailment are caused by virus and the child may need no treatment. You can only get antibiotics if the symptoms persists. You can also give the child cold drinks to ease the pains or give him a children's pain killer like paracetamol.

MEASLES

The first symptoms of measles may include a running nose, cough, fever, sore red swollen eyes, small white

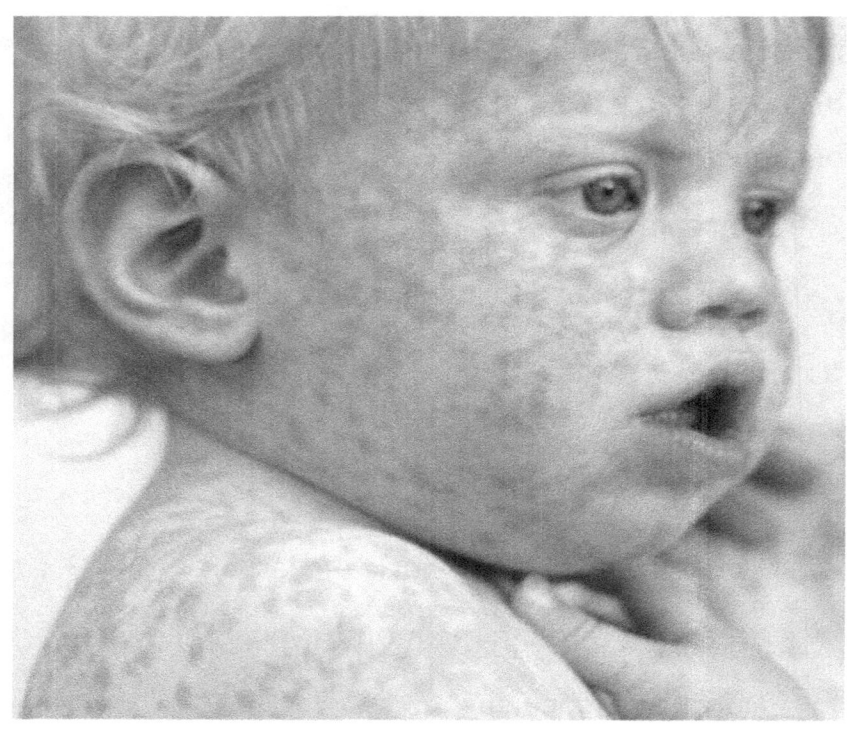

spots in his mouth and a very high fever.

Few days after this symptoms, say like three days, you will begin to notice red behind his ears, on his face and neck. This will spread all over his body and may become bumpy. This rash would be itchy and may last for a few days.

See your doctor immediately you notice the symptoms.

# 26

# BONDING WITH YOUR BABY AFTER BIRTH

Bonding is that feeling you get that makes you want to protect your baby, even with your life. It is a feeling of love you show towards your baby.

Bonding may have occurred even before the birth of the child and you show this love when you talk to your bump.

You may bond immediately with your baby after birth, but if you don't, do not worry about it. But research has that the hormone oxytocin which is released during pregnancy and in large amounts during labour, creates a feeling of euphoria and excitement which makes it easy to love your baby and bond with him immediately.

Even when you have twins, and you don't have access to either of your baby due to one reason or the other, the midwife will encourage you to visit your child wherever he may be to fasten the bonding process.

To make the bonding process fast, let there be skin to skin contact. This can be achieved by placing the child on your chest. With time, the baby will come to know and identify with your smell. Also you should always answer to his cries, hold him close to cuddle, give him plenty of eye contact when he begins to see, smile and talk to him.

Even when you are not holding your baby, always keep him close. Let him always have the feeling that you are around.

Responding to her needs and when she is happy helps to build bonds of trust and tis helps his brain to grow and develop.

Whenever you feel that you are getting tired and can no longer bond with the baby, when you find yourself talking harshly to the baby, try and talk to your doctor or health visitor, you may be suffering from post-natal depression. This depression can lengthen the bonding process. Do not be shy or afraid to talk with your doctor about any feelings you may have towards your baby.

All of these bonding experiences can be experienced by either the father or the mother.

# 27
# GUIDES WHEN TAKING OVER THE COUNTER MEDICINES

Once you are pregnant, you really need to be careful when taking drugs because certain drugs can cause a miscarriage or an adverse effect on the mother and the baby.

It is best not to take over the counter medicines once you are pregnant especially in the first trimester. Advising you not to take over the counter medicines does not mean that there is no remedy to your problem. We are only advising that you take precaution and most importantly see a doctor to make a prescription.

It is quite common to have headaches in the first trimester and you may be tempted to take paracetamol. It may interest you to know that studies have shown a strong link between asthma in children and taking paracetamol during pregnancy. Though more research is needed in this regard, it is better you try and take plenty of water and rest when a bout of headache attacks. Get a doctor's advice before taking that. They would probably advise that you take a minimal dose in the short period of time.

Never take ibuprofen without the advise of your doctor. This has been found to be the leading cause of miscarriages and the common cause of heart diseases in children.

Never take drugs containing codeine except it was recommended by your doctor.

It is common to have indigestion and heartburn problems in the beginning and ending of the pregnancy, especially when the baby becomes big in the tummy pushing up food in your stomach. Meet with your doctor to work out a solution for your indigestion and heartburn.

If you have a stomach upset with diarrhea, never mind, it may be discomforting but it won't harm your baby. Take oral rehydration solutions to take care of your dehydration.

There are many over the counter drugs that would handle your pile if you have one during pregnancy. You can ask the doctor to prescribe one to calm your buttocks.

You won't get thrush medicines over the counter. It is prohibited. Check with your doctor for a prescription.

When you are affected with coughs, colds and flu,

your doctor may use nasal sprays which will not harm your baby. There are other alternatives like inhaling mentholated steam vapor from a bowl of hot water. Honey and lemon in hot water can help soothe your cough.

Talk to your doctor for prescriptions if you have a hay-fever.

# 28

# OTHER FACTORS TO CONSIDER DURING PREGNANCY

There are so many things that you should beware of when you are pregnant. Some of them are discussed in this chapter.

- You should never take aspirin or any non-steroidal anti-inflammatory drugs without the advise from the doctor. This is because it can increase the risk of miscarriage.

- Don't you take alcohol during pregnancy because there is no way to know the right amount of alcohol to take.

- You are advised to have sex regularly during pregnancy because it increases the chance of having a pre-mature baby.

- It is cool to travel by car when you are pregnant as long as you have a healthy pregnancy. If you must drive, then be sure to only drive when you are feeling highly alert and well-rested.

- You should never have electrolysis during pregnancy, it just may harm the child.

- It is completely safe to travel by air if your pregnancy is straightforward and you are feeling very healthy. The safest time to fly is before 37 weeks and 32 weeks if you are expecting a twin.
- It is good to swim during pregnancy. It is a good exercise when you are pregnant.
- You should never smoke during pregnancy. Smoking reduces the oxygen in your cells and may harm the baby.
- Avoid hot weather or places that make you feel very hot.
- It is not safe to have a tattoo during pregnancy.
- Soft mould-ripened cheeses are not good for you during pregnancy, it may have been contaminated by bacteria. If you must eat cheese, take hard, blue-veined cheeses.
-  So long as you cook your seafood very properly, you can eat them since many are safe to eat during pregnancy. They have health benefits for you and your baby.
- Never engage in sports with a high risk of fall or bounce.
- Stay away from hot baths, hot tubs and saunas. A

warm bath is okay.

- Never take over the counter medicines without checking with your doctor first.
- Use a sunscreen whenever you are in sun-bathing.
- Do not engage in scuba-diving. This can lead to decompression sickness which could harm your baby.
- Caffeine intake will not harm your baby. However you are advised to cut down to if you take more than 200milligram a day. Taking more than required amount may lead to miscarriage.
- It is safe to have a leg or bikini wax when you are pregnant.
- It is safe to use essential oils when you are pregnant especially when you are healthy and are careful with them.
- There is no evidence that using a hair bleaching product can harm your pregnancy.
- It is also safe to use relaxers to straighten your hair when you're pregnant, but be sure to note the chemical components of the relaxer before using.

- There is no serious risk of using your mobile phones during pregnancy according to researchers.
- Avoid anything or electronic that raises your temperature over a long period of time. This has the possibility of causing a miscarriage.
- It is not advisable to paint during pregnancy since it would expose you to chemicals.
- If you must use henna, you must make sure that the product is safe, especially when using it as a skin dye.
- Never smoke weed during pregnancy because it can adversely affect the child.
- You can have anal sex during pregnancy if you have a healthy pregnancy. Same for oral sex.
- Never should you eat liver or liver products like liver sausage while you are pregnant or trying to be pregnant because liver contains a very amount of retinol, which may be harmful to your baby.
- It is safe to have the seasonal flu jab when pregnant.
- You can wear tights when you are pregnant.

- You can use sex toys but make sure they are free of disease causing germs.
- You can eat cured meat during pregnancy.
- You can eat pizza as long as they are cooked thoroughly.
- You can take green tea.
- You can use asthma inhalers during pregnancy.
- Depending on the amount of radiation and the type of x-ray, it is safe to have a x-ray during pregnancy.
- Be careful when changing the cat litter during pregnancy to avoid being infected with toxoplsmosis.
- You can use insect repellents with caution during pregnancy.
- Do not varnish wood during pregnancy.
- Acne medicines will harm your baby, do not take them during pregnancy.
- You can use a computer during pregnancy.
- You can use flea sprays during pregnancy.
- You can have acrylic nails during pregnancy.
- It is safe to remove hair removal creams but they

may irritate your skins because of the chemical's reaction to your changing hormones.

- Aerosols and air fresheners contain volatile organic compounds, so it is not advisable to use them routinely during pregnancy.
- It is safe to use a car seat belt when pregnant.
- It is safe to eat pre-washed salads.
- Never eat any uncooked or undercooked meals.
- Keep your high heels away when you are pregnant.
- It is advisable to take folic acid and vitamin D during pregnancy. It is essential for the development of the baby.
- It is not safe to go on a diet when you are pregnant.
- You can have artificial sweeteners during pregnancy but try to have them in moderation.

# RESOURCES

# GLOSSARY

# INDEX

www.ingramcontent.com/pod-product-compliance
Lightning Source LLC
Chambersburg PA
CBHW070305230526
45470CB00002B/729